Judo: Seven Steps to Black Belt
(An Introductory Guide for Beginners)

"Direct, simple, and everything one needs to start off on the right foot in learning judo. I highly recommend this book for anyone serious about learning judo." -- HAYWARD NISHIOKA, 9th degree judo black belt, former national and Pan-American champion, author of several judo books, and two-time Judo Hall of Fame member

"A roadmap for the development of judo expertise, and a valuable review of the foundations of the sport for more advanced practitioners and teachers. I will add many of the descriptions and explanations to my own teaching of judokas at all levels." --CHARLES MEDANI, M.D., 7th degree judo black belt and President of Shufu Judo Yudanshakai, the black belt association of the Mid-Atlantic region of the United States

"People who are considering which martial art to choose for their children, or themselves, should definitely read this book! As a lifelong judoka and father of two judo black belts, I wholeheartedly recommend this book." --ROBERT WINSTON, Colonel, USAF, Retired and 5th degree judo black belt

Judo
Seven Steps to Black Belt

An Introductory Guide for Beginners

Rodolfo Tello

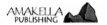
AMAKELLA
PUBLISHING

Disclaimer: The contents of this book are provided for informational purposes only and are not meant to be a substitute for actual judo instruction. The publisher and author of this book assume no responsibility for involuntary errors or omissions, and shall not be liable for any direct or indirect damages that may arise from the practice of judo or out of the use of the data provided in this book. Readers should seek the advice of a qualified medical professional before engaging in judo practice.

Library of Congress Control Number: 2015921059

ISBN-10: 1-63387-001-4
ISBN-13: 978-1-63387-001-7

Cover Design: Línea Digital SAC
www.lineadigital.com

Photographs: 123RF / Fotolia

Amakella Publishing
Arlington, Virginia
www.amakella.com

Printed in the United States of America

CONTENTS

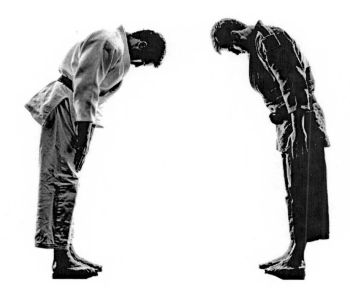

Judo sessions start and end with a bow (rei)

Introduction

Introduction

In ancient Japan, the practice of martial arts experienced exceptional levels of development and diversity. These expressions flourished with the rise of the samurai, sophisticated warriors and elite members of Japanese society. The way of life of the samurai included training in a series of martial art disciplines. Jujitsu was one of them.

In the nineteenth century, however, the changes in Japanese society created a situation in which martial arts had lost a significant part of the prestige and practical use they once enjoyed. By then, Japanese society demanded a new approach to martial arts, no longer focused on the efficient killing of enemies, but rather on the defeat of opponents for sport, self-defense, moral discipline, and personal improvement.

It is in this context that Jigoro Kano, who later became the founder of judo, embarked on a quest to find the most efficient use of mental and physical energy to force opponents into submission. He analyzed the underlying principles behind the different techniques taught in jujitsu and other disciplines, and selected the most efficient of them. He referred to the resulting collection of principles and techniques as judo, to differentiate it from jujitsu, its main predecessor (Kano 2013: 16).

In 1882, Jigoro Kano founded the Kodokan Institute in Tokyo, which started the growth of judo. Today, judo is an Olympic sport practiced by millions of people all over the world. From preschoolers to septuagenarians, judo is practiced for a variety reasons, including sport, self-defense, fitness, character development, recreation, and art, among others. Judo is not only a sport but also a way of life.

Since judo's inception, a key principle of the discipline has been maximum efficiency with minimal effort (seiryoku zenyo). One practical application is that when facing stronger opponents, the recommended action is to temporarily give way instead of offering direct resistance, moving out of the line of attack and getting the opponent off-balance first, and then use that moment to apply a judo technique. That way, the resistance of the opponent will be greatly diminished, and the judo practitioner (judoka) will only need a smaller amount of energy to defeat an opponent.

Seiryoku zenyo is also consistent with many basic principles in physics. If an opponent comes with a great impulse — with the intention of hitting you with a fist, for instance — as a judo practitioner you can take advantage of that inertial movement. You can move into a position favorable to block and grab the attacker's arm, and place your body and hips in a position where they can act as a fulcrum, which together with a lifting movement facilitates the execution of a throw. As Kano stated, "For the purpose of throwing an opponent the principle of leverage is sometimes more important than giving way" (2013: 18).

Action and reaction is another important principle in judo. When we push a person, there is an instinctive tendency for that person to push back in the opposite direction. If we were to pull, the person would likely pull back to return to the original position. Judokas take advantage of those moments when people are moving back to their original position and add their own strength to those movements to apply a technique.

Another example of the application of seiryoku zenyo during sparring (randori) is moving forward and backward (shintai) or in a sliding movement (tai sabaki) to avoid a frontal attack. Repositioning the body in a fluid way, while keeping your center of gravity in balance, can create a moment of confusion when an attacker does not find its intended target where it was supposed to be. In that moment of confusion, an attacker is more vulnerable and exposed, and that moment is usually enough for a judoka to apply a technique and win the confrontation.

The principle of using maximum efficiency with minimal effort allows judo practitioners to throw opponents that are physically bigger and stronger. Instead of risking a frontal attack with uncertain outcomes, it encourages us to get our opponents off-balance first, and then apply judo techniques in a way that requires a smaller amount of energy than frontal confrontations, keeping some energy in reserve for other potential needs.

This general principle applies not only to judo. Seiryoku zenyo can also be applied to many everyday situations outside the mat (tatami). As authors Thompson and Jenkins (2013) pointed out, judo principles can be used in areas like business negotiations, conflict resolution, management strategies, workplace relations, law enforcement, persuasive communications, etc.

Another important principle in judo practice is safety. Judokas need to develop a situational risk awareness to identify potentially dangerous situations for others and ourselves, and make a personal commitment to take preventive measures to decrease the likelihood of such risks from happening and, when unavoidable, to reduce their level of impact. This attitude should be consistent inside and outside the dojo, adopted as a key element in our lives, to create and reproduce a training environment that is both safe and enjoyable for every judo practitioner.

Safety can be greatly enhanced by adopting a precautionary attitude. If we suspect that a risk is imminent, or identify risky situations in which it is probably just a matter of time until they happen, we can take measures to prevent, reduce, and mitigate their negative impact. Examples include identifying potentially dangerous spots at the judo center, and assessing risky behaviors in ourselves and others. Once we identify such areas of risk, we need to say or do something about it.

There used to be situations, particularly in competitions, where continuing to fight after being injured in a match, for instance, was encouraged and praised as an example of a good fighting spirit. However, this attitude in many cases led to situations that placed competitors in greater danger. As a result, the judo community has nowadays adopted a more safety-conscious approach. The case of potential concussions when judokas hit their heads illustrates a situation where, if the potential danger is clearly recognized even without clear symptoms or signs, a judoka must stop competing right away and start resting, favoring a smooth and uneventful recovery process. If the athlete keeps competing, on the other hand, the situation may get much worse and need urgent medical attention, intensifying the problem and potentially keeping the judoka away from judo for a significant period. Remember that safety comes first, and when in doubt, use a precautionary approach, identifying potentially dangerous situations and taking actions aimed at preventing or reducing their impact. Greater care of the judoka is now at the center of judo training courses such as the Heads Up program of the Centers for Disease Control and Prevention, and the Safe Sport course developed by the United States Olympic Committee.

Another key principle in judo is mutual benefit (jita kyoei), intended to develop trust and provide mutual assistance to bring prosperity for the self and others. A direct application of this principle is in the relationship between the partners involved in the practice of judo, where the person performing a technique (tori) requires the presence of a partner (uke) in order to practice and improve such technique.

Being considerate to our fellow judokas is an important part of the judo experience. Once our physical strength and technical skills improve, we need to be careful in the way we use our techniques, according to the level of ability of our partners. If a more advanced judoka were to apply full strength against a novice practitioner, performing several hard throws during a randori (sparring) session, the experience for the novice may not be pleasant, and the person may even consider quitting, leaving the more advanced person with no one to throw next time. Being considerate, and controlling our performance, can allow less skilled judokas to practice their throws, and we can adjust our level of resistance so that they can also learn. This process is more likely to provide a fulfilling experience and contribute to the development of a stronger community of judokas that support each other.

The principle of jita kyoei (mutual benefit) goes beyond the practice of judo. The business philosophy of Konosuke Matsushita, the founder of Panasonic, also illustrates the idea that obtaining benefits for ourselves while benefiting others is a sound approach. He viewed the preference of the public for his business as something entrusted by society, generating an implicit obligation to contribute to "the development of society and the improvement of people's lives" (Panasonic 2015).

Jita kyoei also provides guidance on the type of relationship we should establish with those we regularly interact with in places like home, school, the workplace, the venue where we regularly practice judo (dojo), and even in judo competitions. Jita kyoei promotes different values than the ones adopted by those who advocate winning at all costs, particularly in the context of judo competitions. As Olympic coach and psychology professor David Matsumoto (2003: 16) pointed out, we need to keep in mind that judo is more than winning medals.

This brings us to the issue of judo as a social sport. Judo is not only an end in itself but also a means to achieve higher social and community goals (Figueroa 2004). In the case of judo practice on at-risk children, a study in California found positive effects of judo as part of a community organization program to redirect children's energy away from delinquency and crime in a low-income area. Other studies also identified great potential for a reduction in aggressiveness with judo training. Likewise, studies about the effects of judo practice on the physical and psychological development of handicapped children indicated significant improvements, in which interactions with other judo players helped children deal with problems without force or aggression, acquire coping skills, and become more socially adaptive in general (Imada et al. 2004).

The International Council of Sport Science and Physical Education also highlights the benefits of sport and physical activity in post-disaster interventions. Judo could also be of significant help in support of educational programs, contributing to the development of values such as respect, discipline, and perseverance. The practice of judo promotes teamwork, leadership, and self-confidence, and it can also help prevent issues such as bullying, harassment, aggression, and discrimination. As Matsumoto pointed out, the ultimate goal of judo training is "to develop oneself and one's character so that someday one could improve society and the lives of others" (2003: 17).

The case of Majlinda Kelmendi from Kosovo also illustrates the implications of judo in society. As journalists Morley and Hussain (2015) describe it, "When Majlinda Kelmendi carries her country's flag at the 2016 Olympics, her powerful fighter's shoulders will also bear the weight of expectation of a nation finally gaining recognition after being ripped apart by war." Kayla Harrison's Fearless Foundation, which seeks to enrich the lives of survivors of child sexual abuse through education and sport, is another example of the ways judo can help make a difference in society.

With these considerations in mind, it is time to turn to the more specific treatment of judo techniques. However, the following are some important aspects to take into account before we start learning about the different techniques available in judo:

❖ Judo includes a wide repertoire of techniques, which are important for a greater understanding of the underlying principles of judo. However, some of them are not allowed in competition (shiai), except when they are part of kata, a collection of techniques executed in a predefined sequence. The techniques that are currently not allowed in judo competitions are those that involve touching or grabbing the legs or pants of an opponent from a standing position, which causes the immediate disqualification (hansoku make) of the judo competitor. Grabbing the legs during the matwork part of the competition (ne waza), on the other hand, is perfectly appropriate.

❖ Grappling techniques include holds, chokes and armbars. However, for safety reasons, choking techniques (shime waza) are only allowed for people who are 13 years old or older, and armbars are usually not allowed for people under the age of 16, except in competitions that have a Cadet category, where armbars are allowed at the age of 15.

❖ Traditional jujitsu included joint lock techniques (kansetsu waza) against many joints of the body, including knees, ankles, wrists, fingers, shoulders, spine, and neck, among others. However, the

International Judo Federation (IJF) rules restrict the use of locks against any parts of the body except elbows. Accordingly, this book only refers to the part of kansetsu waza that pertains to armbars.

❖ During your judo studies, you will get exposure to many techniques (waza), which you learn in a gradual way, moving from simple to complex. Eventually, you will develop a preference for some particular techniques, defining favorite techniques (tokui waza) based on their degree of effectiveness (alone or in combination), their level of vulnerability to counterattacks, your individual aptitudes, and your level of technical skill, among other factors.

❖ The techniques that are regularly taught at judo clubs are mostly those used in regular randori, competition, and promotional examinations, but there are many other techniques that are not regularly taught, mostly for safety considerations. Some of the restricted techniques, however, can be safely practiced in the form of kata. Judokas interested in the practice of kata may find it useful to review other books such as the one authored by Kano (2013) and the one by judo experts Otaki and Draeger (1983).

Understanding these factors can help judokas plan a better strategy in the acquisition and later development of their techniques.

Judo techniques fall within two main groups: throwing techniques (nage waza) and grappling techniques (katame waza). While these techniques may be confusing at first, you will gradually become comfortable with them.

A. Throwing techniques (nage waza)

   1. Standing techniques (tachi waza)

      ❯ Hand techniques (te waza)
      ❯ Hip techniques (koshi waza)
      ❯ Foot and leg techniques (ashi waza)

   2. Sacrifice techniques (sutemi waza)

      ❯ Rear sacrifice techniques (ma sutemi waza)
      ❯ Side sacrifice techniques (yoko sutemi waza)

B. Grappling techniques (katame waza)

   1. Holding techniques (osaekomi waza)
   2. Choking techniques (shime waza)
   3. Armbar techniques (kansetsu waza)

More advanced judokas also learn striking techniques (atemi waza) as part of the practice of kata. The glossary included at the end of the book can help you remember unfamiliar terms. The specific techniques in each of these groups will be explained in greater detail in a later chapter. However, before we do that, it is important to review some important topics in preparation for a successful judo experience, providing you with the necessary tools for the early adoption of good habits, paving the way for a safe and enjoyable judo journey, all the way to black belt.

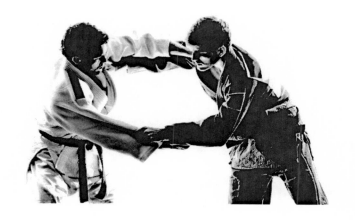

Grip fighting (kumi kata)

Fundamentals of Judo

Fundamentals of Judo

The way we practice judo reflects the type of person we have become. Accordingly, establishing a solid foundation is a key component that shapes subsequent stages in both judo and life, avoiding bad habits that are oftentimes hard to eliminate. Judo can help in the development of good habits from the beginning, so it is worth giving proper consideration to the way we approach judo. The practice of judo can instill positive values, derived from principles such as jita kyoei (mutual assistance to bring prosperity for the self and others), seiryoku zenyo (maximum efficiency with minimal effort), and safety. The practical application of these principles helps us understand what judo is about, and in the process, serves as a guide in our daily decision-making processes. A brief account of Judo etiquette provides an opportunity to illustrate these values and their associated behavior in greater detail.

Judo Etiquette

Judo sessions start with a bow (rei) and end with a bow. The bow is a symbol of respect for our instructors, fellow judokas, the founder of judo, and the judo training area itself. Bowing every time we enter and exit the mat area (dojo) represents a commitment to adhere to the rules of judo and treat people with respect. It is also a symbol of humility and willingness to learn from our instructors and fellow judo practitioners, which helps create a productive training environment.

At the very beginning and at the end of every class, we bow to the image of Jigoro Kano, the founder of judo, who embodies the values and character of a judo practitioner (judoka). By doing so, we acknowledge his contributions and the fact that he dedicated his life to the discipline, developing judo as a carefully designed series of activities that we can practice and benefit from today. We also bow to our instructors to indicate our willingness to learn from them, and to acknowledge their efforts to teach judo to the class. The bow is also an implicit recognition that we will adhere to the specific rules set by the head instructor of our training center (dojo), an expression of trust, and an acknowledgement on the part of the instructor indicating a willingness to share his/her knowledge with the students. The bow also serves as a friendly greeting upon arrival to the class and before departure from the dojo.

Bowing to fellow judokas is also a signal of respect and an expression of willingness to undertake actions leading to our mutual welfare. It is an implicit reminder that a judoka must be careful to prevent injuries to a partner, even when conducting activities such as randori and competition, reducing the risk of injuries during judo matches. Bowing is also an expression of willingness to share what you have learned with other less experienced judoka, helping them improve their techniques, in the same way you would expect more advanced judokas to help you.

Judo etiquette also implies a personal commitment to be perseverant in the practice of judo, and to conduct our activities with safety considerations in mind for ourselves and others. We need to make sure that we do not wear hard or metallic objects that could harm others in class. Our nails should be clipped short to avoid accidental scratches and broken nails. Our judo uniforms (judogis) should be washed after every class.

We also need to avoid performing techniques that could be harmful to our training partners, controlling our throwing attempts so that we do not lose balance and fall on top of our fellow judokas, or allow them to get injured due to our loss of control of their bodies. We also need spatial awareness, stopping when we get close to the limits of the mat, or when we drift close to younger judokas, since we do not want to step on others behind us, or throw our partners on top of nearby players. Likewise, we need to avoid actions that may be harmful for ourselves, such as landing on our heads or arching our backs to prevent our partners from scoring points. Some rules issued by the International Judo Federation (IJF) seek to discourage dangerous actions by penalizing them in competition, but a safety approach should be adopted by every judoka from day one, as a personal commitment inside and outside the dojo.

The Judo Uniform

There are two main types of judo uniforms: single-weave and double-weave. Single-weave uniforms are more suitable for children and teenagers growing at a fast rate. For adults, the recommended type is a double-weave judogi. They are more expensive than single-weave uniforms, but the investment is worth it because of the increased durability, reliability, and performance during training and competition. Women are expected to wear a T-shirt under their judogi, but men should not.

The only colors recognized by the IJF are white and blue. While the Kodokan Institute only accepts white judogi, most judo practitioners around the world use both white and blue uniforms for regular judo practice. In the United States, the minimum recommended number of judogis is two, one white and one blue, since in some high-level tournaments it is required to have both colors for competitions. There are also judogis specifically designed for high-level competition, which must comply with certain requirements established by the IJF.

A big issue with acquiring the right judogi is sizing. As a general rule, all double-weave judogis shrink when washed in hot water and placed into the dryer with a hot setting. Under these conditions, even judogis advertised as pre-shrunk and those whose descriptions state that they will not shrink can have significant shrinkage. Blue judogis tend to shrink a little less than white ones, because they already experienced some degree of shrinking during the dyeing process. Accordingly, there are two approaches to deal with this issue: the first one, which is the one recommended by the manufacturers and many judokas, is to buy a judogi that is only slightly bigger than your size, particularly when it comes to the length of the arms, and then wash it in cold water and hang dry it. There may still be some shrinkage, but it should be minimal, depending on the thickness of the model and the quality of the material.

The second option is to buy a judogi that is one full size bigger than the one you actually need, and then wash it in hot water and place it in the dryer with a medium temperature setting first. If it is still too big, then you can dry it using a hot setting, checking it every ten minutes or so. This treatment will eventually shrink the judogi, so it is better to do it in a gradual way, because there is a good chance that the judogi may shrink beyond what is needed and become unusable. Shrinking a judogi is risky, but if done properly, it will be significantly more practical, since afterward you can treat judogis as normal laundry, using warm settings without expecting much shrinkage after the initial treatment.

The judo uniform needs to be complemented by a belt (obi), which at the beginning is white. Slippers (zori) are also needed to avoid walking barefoot in areas outside the mat. Kneepads are recommended to protect your knees when they enter in contact with the mat (tatami). Elbow protectors may also be useful in competitions, particularly those made out of neoprene, large enough so that they do not restrict free movement or blood circulation. Knee and elbow pads should be soft. Eventually, you may also consider sports tape to protect your fingers from scrapes, and to keep them together to prevent injuries, particularly during competitions. Some people use mouth guards, and in some cases, it may be also helpful to use neoprene shin protectors to absorb the impact of unintended blows, particularly those carried out by enthusiastic beginning judokas.

Anatomy of a Class

After bowing to the side of the wall where the picture of Jigoro Kano is located, and after bowing to the instructors, there is usually a warm-up period. This is important to condition your body and prepare it for the upcoming exercises. The warm-up period usually involves some calisthenics movements and stretching. Key parts of the body to prioritize include shoulders, elbows, wrists, neck, waist, knees, and ankles. Sometimes there are exercises intended to strengthen your muscles, which not only warm up the body but also help build muscular strength. The warm-up period is usually followed by the practice of breakfalls (ukemi) in several directions.

After the breakfall activities, instructors sometimes provide a demonstration of certain techniques, which also serves as a reminder of previously learned techniques. After that, the class usually practices that technique with a partner in repetitive motions (uchi komi), executing them without throwing, to develop muscle memory. These repetitive techniques can be practiced in a stationary position or in movement, with both partners taking turns.

Once people have had the opportunity to practice their techniques, they are asked to seek a partner to practice free sparring (randori), which is a low-intensity match, where the main goal is to improve one's technique in a realistic context. Defeating opponents in randori should be secondary and not as important as improving your technique. Randori begins in the standing position with the goal of performing throws, but it can evolve into a grappling activity (ne waza).

Ne waza provides class participants with the opportunity to practice their holding, choking, and armbar techniques. Ideally, a judoka should seek other people with similar weights and level of skill to make the experience more productive. The main point to remember in randori practice, however, is that judokas should strive to improve their technique, not just rely on raw force to earn scores.

After ne waza, the class enters into a final stage, with additional activities that your instructors may consider appropriate. When this concludes, judoka line up by rank, with the older and more experienced practitioners standing on the right. From this point on, the instructors may have some announcements for the class, including upcoming events and feedback for the class. Sometimes the instructor asks the class members to adopt a kneeling position (seiza) and meditate for a minute or so (mokuso), which allows practitioners to clear their minds after an intensive session. After that, judokas stand up again and bow to their instructors, to the picture of judo founder Jigoro Kano, and to the mat center on their way out.

Open mat is a common practice, where judokas can stay for an additional amount of time after the class is finished, to practice different activities on their own, such as more repetitions of techniques, kata sequences, and additional ne waza activities, among others. This is also a good time to ask questions to the instructors, if they are still around and available. Judokas can at that point request additional demonstrations of techniques, ask questions, strengthen their muscles, or practice any technique with a partner for a little longer.

Performing a Throw

Judo throws need to be carefully thought out and crafted. Oftentimes the different components come together in an instinctive manner, after some time of practicing basic forms in stationary and moving conditions. However, the process of learning the correct application of judo throws can greatly benefit from understanding the four main components of a throw: establishing a solid grip, getting your opponent off-balance, getting your body into position for a throw, and executing the throw with the different parts of your body in a coordinated way. These components are explained in greater detail below.

1. Establishing a firm grip (kumi kata)

The outcome of a match in competition and randori is nowadays influenced to a great extent by the type of gripping control established on every bout. Grip fights are common, and if one opponent establishes a dominant grip, then that person gains more control and has greater chances of applying a technique in a successful way. The person with the dominant grip can set the direction of the match. The greater the level of control over the grip, the greater the chances of winning. This situation is more evident when a right-handed judoka faces an opponent who is left-handed, for instance, which changes the dynamic of the match and leaves room for the other person to find weaker spots that a judoka may not have practiced in a regular way. If you find yourself in a situation when you feel that you are in a vulnerable situation and that an attack from the other person is imminent, then it is likely that the cause may be related to grip control. Gripping skills are a key part of effective throws, which enable the subsequent steps to be performed in a successful way. Accordingly, gripping is an area that judokas need to develop from the beginning, learning to plan gripping strategies and to adapt your gripping tactics for each opponent. As former Olympian medalist and world judo champion Jimmy Pedro points out, "Gripping is one of the most important and fundamental judo skills ... yet it is the least taught and understood skill of the game" (2007). A useful resource is the DVD *Grip Like a World Champion*, released by Pedro in 2007.

2. Getting your opponent off-balance (kuzushi)

Performing a successful throw, one that achieves maximum efficiency with minimal effort, requires getting your opponent off-balance first. You can get your opponent off-balance in eight directions. If you imagine that your opponent is standing on a square, you can get the person off-balance by pushing or pulling, moving the person to the front, back, sides, and corners. Successful kuzushi requires strength and accuracy, leading our opponent in one direction to create momentum and then applying a technique in the opposite direction with explosive movements. By getting your opponent off-balance, you can gain valuable milliseconds to get yourself in position for a throw, before the other person has time to block your attack or apply countermeasures. Kuzushi is a fundamental component of every throw, and it is also one of the areas where opponents are likely to focus their defensive efforts, establishing a rigid posture to restrict the application of kuzushi. This is why muscular development is important, since the muscles associated with the application of successful kuzushi are usually not as strong as the ones used when executing throws. Accordingly, it is important to remember the biomechanics of each throw, identifying where your opponents are directing their efforts, and determining in which direction you should aim your own attack. You need to get your partner off-balance before moving on to the next stage in the throwing sequence. Without proper kuzushi, the chances of completing a judo throw are significantly reduced.

3. Getting into position (tsukuri)

    Once you manage to get your opponent off-balance, the next step is to get yourself into position for the throw. This has to be a coordinated and fluid movement, which usually requires speed, without releasing the pressure that keeps your opponent off-balance. Key factors when getting into position are accuracy when placing your feet in the desired position, equilibrium, stability, and location of your center of gravity, which for many techniques requires you to flex your legs to lower your body. This coordination of movements is better achieved by performing repetitions of your intended techniques (uchi komi). The more you practice those movements, the more fluid they become, acting in a way that resembles an automatic response, activated almost instinctively in response to an opportunity. As judo experts Watanabe and Avakian explained, "The judoist must react with a conditioned reflex to any situation. It must be an automatic response, since there is no time for thinking the situation through" (1990: 19). The movements to get into position may be simple or complicated, and can be part of single techniques or a combination of more than one. What is important is to envision the position you want to be in, and rehearse it many times so that it is ready when needed. Repetitive rehearsal enables judokas to continually develop their technical skills, and the self-confidence that is usually associated with such awareness.

4. Executing the throw (kake)

Once the previous three actions have been conducted, it is time to execute the throw. The most effective throwing movements are those that are performed in an explosive way, which allow for greater speed and force, which are key components of throws that get awarded an instant winning score (ippon). Scoring an ippon usually requires that our throws end up with our opponents landing on their backs, while we maintain control over the action. The simultaneous and explosive movement of the different parts of the body in a coordinated way is likely to end up in a successful throw, unless the opponent is able to adapt and figure a way out. In cases when only a partial score is achieved as a result of a throw, such as a yuko (when our opponents land on the side of their torso after we perform a throw), once on the ground it is important to continue the rolling motion because it can lead to a higher score, such a wazari (when our opponents land largely on their backs after we perform a throw that lacks power, speed or control). After that, you are also likely to be in an advantageous position to apply a ne waza technique, such as pinning your opponent into the mat, which can then evolve into a choking or armbar technique, particularly if you take advantage of the moment when your opponent tries to break the hold.

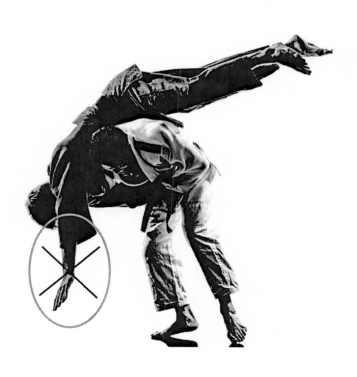

Tori (white) applying a seoi nage technique. Uke should avoid extending his arm to prevent the fall

Judo Techniques

Judo Techniques

The core of judo practice sessions is geared toward learning judo techniques and applying them in practice. After an initial demonstration by an instructor, judo practitioners are expected to perform those techniques, and improve their usage in a gradual way. Repetitions are important to develop muscle memory. The initial emphasis should be on the form of the techniques, and then gradually use them with greater strength, accuracy, and speed. However, first we need to make sure that the form of the movement is correct; otherwise, we risk developing bad habits created by the incorrect application of the different judo techniques.

You gradually acquire a repertoire of techniques, which you can later apply in practice during randori. Some techniques are better suited than others for certain situations, so deciding which technique to use in a particular circumstance is part of a strategy that every judoka needs to develop. The initial tendency is to use those techniques we are more comfortable with, but some situations could be better addressed with techniques we are less familiar with. Balancing your individual strengths with the specific needs of a particular match should be part of a strategy to make the most efficient use of the available resources at your level of skill.

Some strategies to face opponents can be planned in advance, such as when deciding what type of techniques may be better suited for taller opponents, for instance. However, in practice, our initial strategies must be constantly reevaluated and updated for every bout. Oftentimes the definition of a strategy is done instinctively, but if we can develop the habit of planning our strategies and tactics in an intentional way, we are more likely to obtain satisfactory results in a consistent manner.

Technical knowledge of judo is one of the most effective ways of forcing an opponent into submission, and is significantly more important than raw strength alone. However, techniques are most effective when paired with muscular strength and endurance training. Developing a repertoire of judo techniques that you can use in a reliable way and achieving an optimal state of physical conditioning may take a long time, which is why it is recommended that the training of adult judo practitioners should include both technical knowledge and physical development training in parallel.

Since most techniques involve a fluid sequence of different movements, static graphics do not illustrate judo techniques very well. Accordingly, readers are highly encouraged to watch videos demonstrating the application of judo techniques. YouTube® in particular offers a wide selection of techniques, available for free, which can be searched by name or by prearranged series of techniques such as dai ikkyo (first group of techniques) or judo ukemi (breakfalls). Likewise, an organized list of judo techniques in video and animated versions can be found at judoinfo.com. Later on, you may also want to visit judovision.org and ippon.tv to watch the practical application of such techniques in the context of international judo competitions. The following sections describe the main judo techniques organized by groups.

Breakfalls (Ukemi)

Most training centers focus on developing technical skills to perform standing throws (nage waza), which create the need for all judokas to be highly proficient in breakfalls, as the first group of techniques to be practiced and mastered before moving on to learning more advanced ones. Learning and practicing the proper ways to break the falls is important to prevent injuries. Ukemi should be regularly practiced by judo practitioners of all levels.

Breakfalls can be practiced in four directions: backward (ushiro ukemi), forward (mae ukemi), and to the right or left side (yoko ukemi). Breakfalls are also practiced as forward rolling breakfalls (zempo kaiten ukemi or mae mawari ukemi). Forward rolling breakfalls are performed staying down or continuing onto a standing position. Watching the videos of these techniques can help novice judoka get a better sense of their purpose and usage.

Breakfall techniques (ukemi) should be practiced at the beginning of every judo class so that they become part of the subconscious response of the body when it becomes the subject of a throw. When the feet of someone being thrown end up in a position that is way higher than their heads, it may be confusing to know which arm to use, where to direct the mitigating breakfall action, and to time it appropriately to mitigate the fall. However, with regular practice breakfall techniques become increasingly instinctive, accurate, and reliable.

Throwing (Nage Waza)

When it comes to the specific techniques, particularly those required for promotional exams, it is recommended to focus on the throwing techniques within the gokyo no waza group, which comprises 40 techniques, clustered together in five groups, according to the level of experience of the judo practitioner. Key attributes of a throw are force, speed and control.

Beginners should start practicing the eight throwing techniques in the first group (dai ikkyo), and from them move gradually into the more advanced groups.

The throwing techniques included as part of the five groups in the gokyo no waza are the following ones:

1. Dai ikkyo (first group)
   - ➤ Deashi barai
   - ➤ Hiza guruma
   - ➤ Sasae tsuri komi ashi
   - ➤ Uki goshi
   - ➤ Osoto gari
   - ➤ O goshi
   - ➤ Ouchi gari
   - ➤ Seoi nage

2. Dai nikyo (second group)
   - ➤ Kosoto gari
   - ➤ Kouchi gari
   - ➤ Koshi guruma
   - ➤ Tsuri komi goshi
   - ➤ Okuri ashi harai
   - ➤ Tai otoshi
   - ➤ Harai goshi
   - ➤ Uchi mata

The first two groups in the gokyo no waza contain most of the fundamental techniques used in judo. Accordingly, novice judokas should focus on learning those well.

3. Dai sankyo (third group)
   - ➤ Ko soto gake
   - ➤ Tsuri goshi
   - ➤ Yoko otoshi
   - ➤ Ashi guruma
   - ➤ Hane goshi
   - ➤ Harai tsuri komi ashi
   - ➤ Tomoe nage
   - ➤ Kata guruma

4. Dai yonkyo (fourth group)
    - Sumi gaeshi
    - Tani otoshi
    - Hane maki komi
    - Sukui nage
    - Utsuri goshi
    - O guruma
    - Soto maki komi
    - Uki otoshi

5. Dai gokyo (fifth group)
    - O soto guruma
    - Uki waza
    - Yoko wakare
    - Yoko guruma
    - Ushiro goshi
    - Ura nage
    - Sumi otoshi
    - Yoko gake

Learning the purpose and movements associated with each judo technique is a very important part of the training process, including the specific direction of kuzushi for each technique. Understanding when it would be a good time to use each technique is another key area that judokas should strive to understand.

There are also other techniques not included as part of the original gokyo no waza. Some of these more recently accepted techniques (shinmeisho no waza) in the judo repertoire are included next:

> ➤ Hane goshi gaeshi
> ➤ Harai goshi gaeshi
> ➤ Harai maki komi
> ➤ Ippon seoi nage
> ➤ Kouchi gaeshi
> ➤ Ouchi gaeshi
> ➤ O soto gaeshi
> ➤ O soto maki komi
> ➤ Sode tsuri komi goshi
> ➤ Tsubame gaeshi
> ➤ Uchi mata sukashi
> ➤ Uchi mata gaeshi
> ➤ Uchi mata maki komi

Some techniques are more widely used than others. Throwing techniques beginning judokas may want to consider are:

> ➤ Ippon seoi nage
> ➤ Ouchi gari
> ➤ Uchi mata
> ➤ Tai otoshi
> ➤ Sasae tsuri komi ashi

A useful visual resource with detailed explanations and demonstrations of uchi mata, including slow-motion scenes, can be found in a DVD developed by former judo Olympian Israel Hernandez (2015). This video explains in detail the different grips, variations, common mistakes, counters, combinations, and suggested exercises to improve the use of this technique. It can give you an idea of the complexity of tasks involved in the execution of a single technique, which can later be used to approach the study of other techniques with a similar level of detail. Learning about the specificity of uchi mata would be also beneficial for judokas developing their favorite technique (tokui waza).

Grappling (Katame Waza)

Grappling refers, for the most part, to the application of judo techniques once judokas are on the ground, including holding or pinning (osaekomi waza), choking (shime waza), and arm locks (kansetsu waza). Please note the minimum age restrictions for the use of choking techniques (13) and armbars (16), which were previously noted.

Katame waza is closely related to ne waza, but these two terms are slightly different. Ne waza refers only to judo matwork techniques, while Katame waza has a broader scope and includes the application of joint techniques on the ground and from a standing position (Kano 2013: 55). Ne waza, however, is the most commonly used term when referring to grappling techniques. The main three groups of judo techniques in katame waza are:

1. Osaekomi waza (holding techniques)
   - Hon kesa gatame
   - Kuzure kesa gatame
   - Kata gatame
   - Yoko shiho gatame
   - Kami shiho gatame
   - Kuzure kami shiho gatame
   - Tate shiho gatame

2. Shime waza (choking techniques)
  ➤ Nami juji jime
  ➤ Gyaku juji jime
  ➤ Kata juji jime
  ➤ Hadaka jime
  ➤ Okuri eri jime
  ➤ Kataha jime
  ➤ Katate jime
  ➤ Sode guruma jime
  ➤ Ryote jime
  ➤ Tsukkomi jime
  ➤ Sankaku jime

3. Kansetsu waza (armlock techniques)
  ➤ Ude garami
  ➤ Ude hishigi ude gatame
  ➤ Ude hishigi juji gatame
  ➤ Ude hishigi hiza gatame
  ➤ Ude hishigi waki gatame
  ➤ Ude hishigi hara gatame
  ➤ Ude hishigi ashi gatame
  ➤ Ude hishigi te gatame
  ➤ Ude hishigi sankaku gatame

A useful resource for learning competitive applications of judo matwork techniques is the book *Winning on the Ground*, written by judo experts De Mars and Pedro (2013).

Sparring (Randori)

Randori usually starts in a standing position and then it may continue into matwork (ne waza randori). In practice, there are two main types of randori: light and hard. Hard randori is usually practiced when people try to score throws or avoid being thrown, spending lots of energy in the process. This attitude is found among many beginning judokas, even though this approach may be detrimental to their learning process. Hard randori tends to mask weaknesses in the technical abilities of a judoka, who needs to rely on physical strength to compensate for poor technical skills. It also requires high levels of energy, which prevents these judo practitioners from participating in more than a few randori matches, gradually decreasing their level of effectiveness, and often losing by exhaustion.

A light randori approach, on the other hand, is a better option since it allows more flexibility and the use of concentrated strength only during those moments when it is needed, allowing judokas to apply their techniques in better conditions, and last longer with similar levels of energy. By participating in more randori matches on average, judo practitioners get more opportunities to try their techniques. Light randori also offers greater sensitivity to anticipate the attacks of an opponent, and gives you advance warning, particularly in the case of techniques applied poorly and with unnecessary force. It also provides more opportunities to identify moments of vulnerability in our opponents that we can use to settle a match. The combination of this flexible approach, along with short intervals of explosive movements, is more likely to produce successful results on a consistent basis, while also providing a safer and more enjoyable judo experience in general.

Judokas that view randori as an opportunity to improve their technical knowledge of judo will make more progress than the ones that only focus on throwing people, even if that is accomplished by the use of lousy techniques or raw strength. As Judo Hall of Fame member Hayward Nishioka pointed out, "When you come down to it, judo is technique-oriented first. If it were not so, a weight-lifter or a long-distance runner would be world champion in judo" (2000: 19).

It is also important to remember that some judo techniques are forbidden both in competition and in the regular practice of randori. The main reason for such restrictions is the safety of the judokas, since these techniques present a high risk of injury. Some of these prohibited-use techniques are kani basami, do jime, kawazu gake, daki age, and ashi garami.

In addition, all techniques that require touching or grabbing an opponent's leg or pants are now restricted and cannot be used in competition, according to the current rules (as of the date of publication) of the International Judo Federation. These changes restrict the use of techniques such as kata guruma, sukui nage, morote gari, kuchiki taoshi, kibisu gaeshi, and te guruma, among others. Non-standard grips that are not followed by immediate attacks are now also penalized in competition.

On the matter of safety, however, it is important to specify that any technique that is incorrectly applied may pose a risk of injury. Accordingly, judokas should strive to learn judo techniques in a way that is both safe and effective. Particular attention is due to the group of techniques known as maki komi, which may pose a risk of shoulder injury for your opponent when the throw is only halfway completed, creating shoulder-landing situations.

Techniques are more effective and safer when they have been practiced on a continuous basis, because it gives judokas a greater understanding of how they are used under different conditions. It is important to learn well a small group of favorite techniques first, and then expand your repertoire of techniques in a gradual way. Start with one or two techniques that you really want to master first, and then gradually add more techniques. Quality is more important than quantity.

Both randori and competition (shiai) benefit greatly from the use of combinations, particularly when they are part of a sequence of follow-up techniques that a judoka has planned and rehearsed in advance. If the first technique applied faces resistance from an opponent, then we can follow up immediately with a second and third attempt, using other techniques that are best suited to take advantage of the new position of the opponent. The selection of techniques to be used in combination depends on the preferences and level of skill of each person, but the important idea to remember is that we need to identify the different likely scenarios and plan appropriate actions for each of them. When attacking, we should develop the habit of not stopping after the first attempt, but continue trying after that. Examples of combinations of techniques include kouchi gari followed by ippon seoi nage on the opposite side, and kouchi gari followed by ouchi gari and then followed by uchi mata.

Combinations also include the transition from a standing position (nage waza) to matwork (ne waza), particularly when we are placed in a position that favors that transition. Good opportunities usually present themselves after we score a partial throw (yuko or wazari), which create situations when we already have a hold of an arm and are placed in a position where it is easier to move on top of an opponent. Likewise, there are times when we face strong resistance from an opponent in the standing position, so we may want to transition into ne waza to create more opportunities. As Japanese judo champions Inokuma and Sato explained, the use of nage waza techniques alone "might not be enough for a winning score ... be prepared for this and practice daily to master moving from throwing techniques to grappling techniques" (1986: 178).

Randori is at the core of judo, a space where different preparatory actions converge, and consequently, it should be an activity with a high level of priority. Randori should be an area of permanent study, experimenting and reflecting on our effectiveness, as will be further discussed in the next chapter on performance.

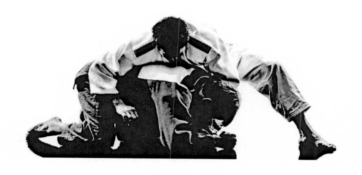

Ne waza

Improving Performance

Improving Performance

The best way to improve performance in judo is by being perseverant in regular practice. Judo offers constant opportunities for improvement, which we can take advantage of by adopting an attitude of constant reflection about our performance. Regardless of how well we did on a particular day, the goal should be to analyze the reasons behind our success, or lack thereof. Instead of focusing just on the outcome of a match, the most important concern should be understanding the reasons and factors leading to a given outcome in the application of judo techniques. This should be a constant effort, leading to greater understanding of the nuances involved in the application of judo techniques.

There are also activities that could be conducted in parallel to improve performance. Physical conditioning can help build the necessary strength for the application of judo techniques, particularly when we face strong judoka that like to assume a defensive position. Psychological preparation is also important to develop the right attitude. Likewise, participating in competitions on a regular basis provides opportunities to get feedback and learn, while also requiring you to pay closer attention to the rules of judo competition. The practice of kata can also contribute in significant ways to the improvement of judo techniques. These activities are briefly discussed next.

Physical Conditioning

Optimal performance in judo requires a good physical condition, which needs to be cultivated over a long period. Key areas that need to be developed in physical conditioning include a combination of endurance and performance training (aerobic and anaerobic exercises), and muscular development.

Developing your muscles is a long-term effort, which needs to be initiated early in the judo training process. The type of activities included as part of the muscular development process will vary. Adults are encouraged to include weightlifting as part of their activities, but younger practitioners should refrain from lifting weights until they reach an appropriate level of physical development. The specific type of exercises to be conducted needs to be determined by both a certified training coach and a medical professional, in addition to your judo instructor, who can help you identify which areas you should focus your efforts. Muscular development should involve the whole body, prioritizing power over muscular mass, and include training of the forearms (for strong grips) and calves (to help lift your opponents), which are sometimes overlooked.

Performance training focuses on the ability to execute high-intensity tasks in a short period of time. Explosive movements are the most effective in judo throws, but they also require spending a great amount of energy. Short sprints, for instance, create the type of response that the body needs to get used to that type of movements in the application of judo techniques. Plyometric exercises are also highly recommended to increase power, which is the combination of speed and strength. Cardiovascular fitness, however, is best achieved when it is the result of a combination of both anaerobic and aerobic exercises, explosive movements, and physical endurance.

Endurance is part of a process that, depending on your overall physical condition, may take weeks or months to achieve. It is a process that people should not try to force in order to make quick progress. The reason is that endurance is closely related to blood circulation, and overstressing your body during exercise could be detrimental to your heart, among other health risks. There are target heart rates that should not be exceeded. As Nishioka explains, judokas can use the Kaiser Permanente formula for determining their target heart rate (THR): Men THR = 220 - athlete's age x 0.65; Women THR = 225 - athlete's age x 0.65 (Nishioka 2010: 93). For further information on this topic, please refer to a specialized resource or consult a healthcare professional.

Aging athletes that took long breaks from judo are particularly at risk of experiencing health issues. They may be eager to go back to their former levels of performance, but this could create pressures that their bodies are not ready to accept before an extended period of physical conditioning. In those cases, it is important to be patient, exercising regularly but at levels that do not exceed their recommended Target Heart Rate, and abstaining from competition until they have been cleared by a physician. Judokas in these circumstances may also need to reevaluate the techniques they practiced in the past, making adjustments as needed.

Once you achieve your desired level of cardiovascular conditioning and muscular development, maintaining a good physical condition should be basically a matter of attending regular judo practice plus a combination of light exercise activities. At least an hour of jogging per week, adjusting it to your convenience, would be a good complement to judo practice, keeping judokas in shape. Flexibility is also important, which is usually achieved and maintained by conducting regular stretching activities when our bodies are warm, particularly before and after judo practice.

Psychological Preparation

The right mental attitude can be a significant factor in a successful judo training experience, which is reflected in the performance of a judoka. As sport psychology authors Ravizza and Hanson explain, consistent preparation and the ability to focus make a big difference in the performance of athletes, particularly when they exercise positive control over their thoughts so that they can deliver the best of themselves, visualizing the successful execution of their moves in their minds, and feeling confident about their ability to perform them in practice (1998). Former judo Olympian Rhadi Ferguson also points out that, beyond physical aspects, being good at judo depends largely on "your ability to think, process, apply and adapt" (2014).

Motivation is a key factor behind a successful performance in judo. Different people have different ways of getting motivated, so you need to find out what motivates you. Some people get motivated by watching videos of top-level judo competitions, reading the personal stories of famous judo figures, or by the idea of getting promoted and moving up in the ranks, among other ways. You need to identify a source of inspiration that works for you.

Determination is another important attribute, which implies the need to follow through with your judo activities on a regular basis. Being consistent in judo practice and other complementary physical preparation activities is an important aspect, along with the desire to keep trying your techniques even when their success is not readily apparent, without getting discouraged in the process.

Proactive behavior is also necessary to make gradual improvements. We cannot adopt a passive attitude or get into the habit of adopting a defensive posture. We need to seek the fight, moving our opponents around and generating the spaces to get them out of balance, so we can perform our throws. The first person that initiates an action sets an anchor that defines the pace and direction of each bout, helping him/her establish control of the match.

Adopting an assertive attitude is also important in the process of improving your performance in judo. There are inner struggles to overcome the different types of challenges involved in the practice of judo, which need to be confronted with self-discipline on a regular basis. As former judo Olympian and mixed martial arts champion Ronda Rousey pointed out, "You have to fight your body when it tells you it is tired. You have to fight your mind when doubt begins to creep in ... to get anything of real value, you have to fight for it" (2015: 2). The mental determination to confront our inner problems in order to win applies not only to judo but to life in general.

Participating in Competition

Competition in tournaments (shiai) is an important part of judo practice. One of the most important benefits of participating in judo competitions is the knowledge you can gain from those experiences, identifying strengths and weaknesses, and using that information to make adjustments to improve your training strategy. Shiai allows judokas to get a feeling of their current level of performance in relation to other judo practitioners that fall into a similar category in terms of weight, age, gender, and level of experience, among other criteria. The best way to get familiar with judo competitions is to attend as many as you can as an observer. You can also watch matches of international tournaments at the IJF's official channel on YouTube.®

A key factor related to competition is learning the rules set by the International Judo Federation. Being aware of what is allowed and what is prohibited during a match is critical, since it could lead to the efficient use of the rules in your favor or to wasted opportunities. Elite competitors are very aware of the rules governing judo competitions, but such knowledge should be present among every judoka participating in competition. Learning the rules of judo competition should be a priority among judokas.

One of the most common mistakes among novice judokas, particularly junior competitors, is that oftentimes they are not familiar with the vocabulary used by judo referees, so when they hear the word "osaekomi," for instance, they release their opponents instead of keeping them pinned to the mat, wasting a valuable opportunity to score points. Osaekomi is the call to start the timer for the hold down. Under current regulations, when competitors keep their opponents pinned for 10 seconds they score a yuko. If they keep them pinned for 15 seconds, they score a wazari, and can even score an ippon (instant win) after 20 seconds. Osaekomi starts the clock, indicating that a competitor has successfully started a pin on an opponent, but lack of knowledge of the meaning of this word and its rules can affect the results of a match in significant ways.

The most important actions leading to light penalties (shido) include non-combativity, defensive position, stepping out of the inner boundaries of the mat, preventing the opponent from establishing a grip, and using non-standard grips that are not immediately followed by an attack. Situations leading to severe penalties (hansoku make) are less common and need to be analyzed in each specific circumstance. The rules of judo competition, however, can be extensive and constantly changing, which is why judokas are encouraged to review the most recent version of the rules by downloading them directly from the website of the International Judo Federation. Judokas are also encouraged to get certified as judo referees once they reach brown belt levels.

Weight management is another important factor in competition. Since athletes who are close to the top limits of their weight categories often have an advantage in terms of strength, judokas who are slightly over the limits of their categories usually try to lose weight before a tournament, so they can fit into their intended category. Accordingly, it is important to develop a strategy for losing weight in a healthy and controlled way. Adjustments in eating habits, measured water intake, and controlled dehydration play a key part in this process, but it is very important to seek the advice of a professional trainer or healthcare professional before implementing a rapid weight loss strategy, since there may be considerable health risks if this process is not performed properly. It is also important to remember that losing weight rapidly usually reduces an athlete's performance in a proportional way, so the more weight you lose, the greater the level of anticipated decrease in performance.

Because of the level of physical stress required, judo competitions require athletes to reach their optimal level of physical performance. If performance were to be affected by recently healed injuries or lack of physical conditioning, it would be advisable to wait until the next tournament when the levels of performance are not diminished by such factors.

One of the best ways to prepare for a competition is the frequent practice of randori. The level of performance of a judoka tends to increase in a proportional level to the time spent in randori practice. For instance, judokas who practice randori for 90 minutes per week are likely to be better positioned to do well in a competition than people who only spend 40 minutes per week in randori. Reflecting on one's performance after every session, and planning the techniques we want to use before every judo session, also help us make significant progress.

The last training days before a tournament usually involve a heavier emphasis on repetitive techniques (uchi komi), focusing just on favorite techniques. You can pick no more than four techniques and rehearse them in static and moving situations, reinforcing your muscle memory. Explosive movements and combinations are also important, since scoring points during tournaments (shiai) usually requires a combination of well-applied techniques, with enough strength and speed, identifying the proper openings to apply the four steps in the execution of a throw: establishing a firm grip, getting your opponent off-balance, placing yourself in a throwing position, and executing the throw. Developing the habit of rolling on the ground, after achieving a partial score such as yuko, is also helpful.

There is also a psychological component to doing well in competition. Knowledge of your own strengths can help you apply your judo techniques with confidence. Knowledge of the rules governing judo competitions is also helpful in acting with confidence. Goal-setting is also important, particularly when you set up realistic indicators to measure success. Judo competitions should not be seen as isolated events but as elements of a larger strategy, leading to the fulfillment of higher goals. Keeping your eyes on the prize will also allow you to keep smaller incidents in perspective.

The Practice of Kata

Kata, the application of a series of judo techniques prearranged in a formal sequence, is an integral part of judo. It allows judo practitioners to gain a better understanding of judo techniques, many of which can be directly used in randori and shiai, allowing judokas to gain a greater understanding and control in the application of judo techniques in general. The katas practiced are representative of the different techniques available in judo.

Rather than a rigid set of movements, kata should be understood as a dynamic and flexible activity. As Otaki and Draeger explain, kata allows judo practitioners to incorporate many principles of martial arts ways, including elements such as "simplicity, natural efficiency, harmony, intuition, economy of movement, and 'softness' of principle that characterizes all traditional Japanese art forms" (1983).

There are many katas in judo. However, the seven judo katas that are currently taught at the Kodokan Institute are the following ones:

1. Nage no kata
2. Katame no kata
3. Kime no kata
4. Goshin jutsu
5. Ju no kata
6. Itsutsu no kata
7. Koshiki no kata

Kata can be practiced by all judokas, including beginners and children. The practice of kata is for the most part optional, except in the case of nage no kata, which is a requirement for promotion to advanced brown belts and black belt. Nage no kata involves the application of hand throwing techniques (te waza), hip techniques (koshi waza), foot and leg techniques (ashi waza), rear sacrifice techniques (masutemi waza), and side sacrifice techniques (yoko sutemi waza).

Kata is usually practiced in the context of formal demonstrations, kata tournaments, and promotional exams, but kata should be understood in a broader context. Katas can be used to teach techniques that would be too dangerous to use in regular randori practice. The coordination skills developed in kata practice are also important, since they can help judoka anticipate the movements of their partners. Overall, the practice of kata can help develop a greater understanding of judo and confidence in the application of judo techniques.

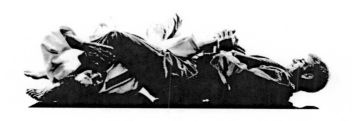

Ude hishigi juji gatame (kansetsu waza)

The Seven Steps

The Seven Steps

We tend to perform better when we set clear goals we want to achieve. For beginning judokas, one such goal is earning a black belt. Traveling the path to achieving that goal is not easy, but having a long-term plan in place can contribute toward that goal in significant ways, helping you place judo in a high position among different priorities in life, which oftentimes have to compete for your limited time and attention.

Progress may not be always steady, since there are many factors that can be detrimental in this process. Recovering from injuries, moving to a place where attending regular judo classes is not practicable, and work scheduling conflicts, for instance, may be factors beyond our control. However, most difficulties are temporary in nature, so sooner or later you may get a chance to resume judo practice, which is why it is important to think about judo as a long-term activity.

Milestones in terms of progress achieved by judo beginners are known as kyu ranks, which are differentiated by belt colors. They follow a ranking system originally developed by Jigoro Kano, and later adopted by other martial arts as well. Each kyu represents the level of achievement and experience of a judoka, but it also implies a responsibility for the judoka to continue improving, to live up to the standards expected from someone at a given rank.

The requirements for moving up in the ranks vary according to each level. This book takes as a reference the promotional standards of the United States Judo Federation, as used by Shufu Yudanshakai (the black belt association of the Mid-Atlantic region). These requirements include general requirements such as moral character, assertive attitude, maturity, technical proficiency, general experience, contributions to the discipline, and time in grade. Competitive ability is also important, except in the case of non-competitors. Each level of achievement is represented here as a step in the long but rewarding process toward the attainment of the black belt level.

The levels described next are only applicable for senior judoka, which is usually a category for judokas who are at least 16 years old. Junior judokas follow a similar sequence but with many more steps in the process, and eventually they have to make a transition to the senior rank system before being established on their path to black belt, which varies according to the organization granting the ranks. The following sections illustrate these levels. However, this information is provided for reference purposes only, since the actual requirements may be different in your region.

First Step: Rokkyu

The first step in the sequence, and one of the most important ones, is starting to practice judo on a regular basis. Judo is a very hands-on activity, so the best way to experience it is to get started, and from that point on continue a process of continuous learning and improvement. New judokas are assigned the rank of rokkyu (sixth kyu) and wear a white belt. This step can last around six months, but the actual time in grade will vary depending on the specific conditions displayed by each individual, as well as the test scheduling practices of each judo club. Some clubs only schedule tests twice a year, for instance, so actual time in grade may vary significantly.

An important part of the initial training process is spent practicing breakfalls (ukemi). Breakfalls should be practiced regularly by judokas of all levels, but are particularly important for beginners. Falling techniques are as important as throwing techniques. During this period, the throwing techniques to learn are the ones specified in the first group (dai ikkyo) of the gokyo no waza: deashi barai, hiza guruma, sasae tsurikomi ashi, uki goshi, osoto gari, o goshi, ouchi gari, and seoi nage (the latter can be performed with techniques such as ippon seoi nage, morote seoi nage and eri seoi nage).

Before moving on to the next level, judokas are expected to successfully perform breakfalls (ukemi), throws from a standing position (nage waza), and grappling techniques (katame waza), and learn basic Japanese terminology used in the practice of judo. The katame waza component usually requires a demonstration of the following techniques: hon kesa gatame, kata gatame, yoko shiho gatame, and kami shiho gatame.

In addition to regular judo practice, it is recommended to review the written materials developed by the judo organization in your region (yudanshakai), which may have produced guidance documents outlining the specific expectations for each rank. Judo etiquette questions and judo history may also come up in the promotional tests, so it is important to assign enough time for adequate preparation. Books are very helpful in this process. A list of the top seven resources I recommend is included at the end of the book.

Second Step: Gokyu

After successfully completing the testing requirements for the first level, senior judokas are granted the rank of gokyu (fifth kyu), represented by a green belt, according to the coloring system used by the United States Judo Federation. The expectations for judokas at this level are higher, including a greater emphasis on the technical side of judo techniques.

If a judoka has not started working on muscular development yet, this is the time to start doing it. Physical conditioning may take a long time to achieve, so it is important to get an early start. This is also a good time to begin participating in competitions to get experience, with some basic knowledge to apply judo techniques in a successful way, and early enough in the process to start receiving useful feedback to incorporate in the learning process.

In addition to the knowledge of the judo techniques for the previous level, judokas holding the level of gokyu should also learn the second group of techniques (dai nikyo) of the gokyo no waza: harai goshi, kosoto gari, kouchi gari, koshi guruma, okuri ashi harai, tai otoshi, tsuri komi goshi, and uchi mata. Likewise, the promotion test will likely include the following katame waza techniques: kuzure kesa gatame, kuzure kami shiho gatame, and tate shiho gatame, in addition to choking techniques (shime waza), and combinations (renraku waza). Judokas who are at least 16 years old are also required to perform arm locks (kansetsu waza). Other general judo skills likely to be tested for the next level include different breakfalls (ukemi), establishing a firm grip (kumi kata) in randori, getting your partner off-balance (kuzushi), general posture and attitude (shisei), and the general movement of the body (shintai and tai sabaki). Time in grade before promotion varies, but the minimum expected time would be three to six months of regular judo practice.

Third Step: Yonkyu

After completing the basic requirements and achieving the level of skill necessary to perform the judo techniques expected for judokas wearing a green belt, judo practitioners can test for the next level (yonkyu), which is represented by a blue belt, according to the coloring system used by the USJF.

Blue belt is the optimal time to compete in judo tournaments. At this level, a judoka already has developed the necessary knowledge of randori for an effective application of throwing and grappling techniques, and has a significant enough understanding of judo to do well in a tournament. At this point, the level of skill of judokas normally allows them to engage in competitions in a more technically robust manner than before, in safer conditions than someone who just began in judo, and face higher-ranking judoka as well.

In addition to the accumulated knowledge of the judo techniques required for the previous levels, judokas holding the level of yonkyu (blue belt) should learn the third group of techniques (dai sankyo) of the gokyo no waza: ko soto gake, tsuri goshi, yoko otoshi, ashi guruma, hane goshi, harai tsuri komi ashi, tomoe nage, and kata guruma. Judokas at this level should also learn different techniques of defense and escape on the mat (katame waza), including osaekomi waza (holding), shime waza (choking), and kansetsu waza (armbars).

The minimum time in grade as a blue belt (yonkyu) is six months, but in practice, it may vary significantly, since many people at this level tend to avoid testing until they can further improve their judo skills. However, the general recommendation is not to wait for too long, since in the process of preparing for a promotion test a judoka usually allocates more time to study and reflect on the principles and techniques of judo, improving his/her knowledge in the process. Since theory and practice are closely related in the progression of a judoka, the study of judo will be eventually reflected in performance. At this level, the promotional exams usually include both oral and written tests, in addition to the practical demonstration of different types of techniques.

Fourth Step: Sankyu

After a successful test, judokas earn the grade of sankyu and start wearing a brown belt. This may be confusing at first, because there are three levels of brown belt. Accordingly, from this point forward it is better to switch from the color code of the belts to the Japanese terminology used for judo ranks.

In addition to the accumulated knowledge of the judo techniques for all the previous levels, judo practitioners with the grade of sankyu should learn the fourth group of techniques (dai yonkyo) of the gokyo no waza: sumi gaeshi, tani otoshi, hane maki komi, sukui nage, utsuri goshi, o guruma, soto maki komi, and uki otoshi.

The sankyu level is also a period in which a judoka should start getting involved in the regular practice of judo kata, the formal expression of judo techniques prearranged in sequences. For non-competitors (usually people over 35 years old), minimum time in grade is around nine months. Judoka at this level must learn the first three sets of the nage no kata as both uke and tori. Competitors do not have a minimum time in grade; they only need to complete the required number of points before being eligible to test for promotion. Competitors are usually required to perform at least the first three sets of the nage no kata as uke before their next promotion.

Fifth Step: Nikyu

Once promoted, the next level in the judo learning process is nikyu, in which judokas continue wearing a brown belt. In addition to the accumulated knowledge of the judo techniques for all the previous levels, judoka with the grade of nikyu should learn the fifth group of techniques (dai gokyo) of the gokyo no waza: osoto guruma, uki waza, yoko wakare, yoko guruma, ushiro goshi, ura nage, sumi otoshi, and yoko gake.

The minimum time in grade for non-competitors is twelve to eighteen months, depending on the age of the judoka. For people who are 35 years old or more, the time requirements are usually lower. Judokas at this level are expected to learn the complete nage no kata (five series) as both uke and tori. Competitors are usually expected to perform the complete nage no kata as tori before their next promotion. Time in grade for competitors follow different criteria, and could be as little as three to six months if enough competition points are accumulated. For a more detailed explanation of the point system, please refer to the guidance documents issued by the organization under which the testing is done.

At this level, judokas could greatly benefit from the process of getting certified as a judo coach and/or assistant instructor. The learning process involved in the certification process (which could be done by attending specialized clinics or completing distance-learning programs) provides important knowledge that can help judokas improve their judo performance, and prepare them to advise others who are just starting out in judo as well.

Sixth Step: Ikkyu

After completing the requirements and passing the necessary tests, judokas earn the level of ikkyu, the last level in which judo practitioners wear a brown belt. In addition to the accumulated knowledge of the judo techniques for all the previous levels, judo practitioners with the grade of ikkyu should learn all 40 techniques of the gokyo no waza, in addition to osaekomi waza (holding), shime waza (choking), kansetsu waza (armbars), kaeshi waza (counters) and renraku waza (combinations). All techniques should be performed with high levels of precision and control, demonstrating a greater understanding of the biomechanics of a throw, particularly the forces acting in the process of getting uke off-balance before applying a judo technique (kuzushi).

For non-competitors, the minimum time in grade may be eighteen to twenty-four months, depending on the age of the judoka. Non-competitors usually have to learn to demonstrate the complete nage no kata as uke and tori, as well as the katame no kata as uke. Competitors are usually required to perform the complete nage no kata as uke and tori. Time in grade for competitors could be as low as three to six months if enough competition points are earned.

Ikkyu is a level in which judokas should learn more about the rules of competition, and ideally, become certified as judo referees. The certification process provides a great learning opportunity. It usually involves the study of judo regulations, watching videos, participating in clinics, and gaining practical experience at your local judo club and in judo tournaments. For competitors, the knowledge gained can help you become more confident in tournaments and plan a more informed competition strategy, taking advantage of scoring opportunities and avoiding penalties. In some cases where results are very close, the knowledge of the rules can make a difference between winning and losing a match. This knowledge would be also useful when coaching and helping other less experienced judokas prepare for competitions.

Seventh Step: Shodan

The seventh step requires passing the tests to achieve the black belt rank (shodan), which is the first of the advanced levels in the practice of judo. This test is more rigorous and extensive than the previous ones, and usually lasts a full day. There is usually an oral and written test, in addition to a demonstration of all the judo techniques previously discussed.

Earning a black belt level is not the end of the process but the beginning of a new stage. After earning the rank of shodan there are still nine more levels, each of them more demanding than the previous one. Upon achieving the black belt level, judokas usually focus on learning more about judo so that they can teach others the correct application of techniques, creating greater awareness and contributing to the development of judo, and often volunteering for different judo-related activities organized by their clubs and regional black belt associations. Judokas continue the process of learning different katas, including katame no kata and kime no kata. They also focus on improving their teaching skills so that they can assist the head instructor of their dojo in class, as needed.

If inclined to do so, judokas holding the rank of shodan can open their own judo clubs and have them recognized by their regional and national organizations, becoming instructors and managers of their own training centers. The opportunities are many, but the most important thing to remember is that a black belt is only one step along the way in the judo learning process, as part of a continuous progression that should never stop. Understanding that after earning a black belt there is still much to learn, and that there may always be someone stronger and more skilled than us, should be part of the motivation to continue improving. As judo expert Neil Ohlenkamp pointed out regarding the meaning of a black belt, "The belt is not as important as the lessons learned along the way ... a Judo rank is a recognition of accomplishment, but it is the education and training itself that is important ... Black belts are often ordinary people who try harder and don't give up."

The role of judo in shaping character is another important area in which black belt holders can focus their efforts, making judo not only an end in itself but also a means to improve people's lives. As Jigoro Kano pointed out regarding judo as a physical education activity, its aim is "making the body strong, useful and healthy while building character through mental and moral discipline" (2013: 20). The practice of judo can bring people together and help its practitioners reach their potential in life. Black belt holders are in a privileged position to help others bring these goals about, and carry on the judo legacy for mutual benefit and prosperity.

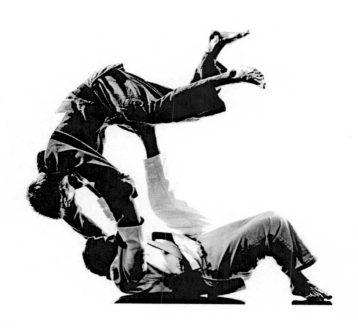

Tomoe nage (sutemi waza)

Final Remarks

Final Remarks

The issues presented in this book address the most common questions posed by beginning judo practitioners. Following the guidelines and recommendations included here can help beginning judoka establish a solid foundation. However, judo is a much broader discipline with many topics and can be a lifetime learning enterprise, which is why it is important to continue learning from other sources. As Nishioka pointed out, judo is "a microcosm of life" (2000: 15), which includes philosophical, spiritual, social and cultural dimensions.

An important step when starting the practice of judo is to join a national organization, such as the United States Judo Federation (USJF), which provides its members with insurance benefits and promotion opportunities. Since judo is a long-term activity, it is highly recommended to choose a life membership, which offers significant benefits. USJF has regional black belt associations, known as yudanshakai, which usually organize tournaments, clinics, and promotional events. Other judo organizations in the United States include USA Judo (USJI), which focuses on the development of judo athletes for national and international competitions, and the United States Judo Association (USJA).

Judo belts reflect the learning commitment and experience level of a judoka, but the learning process sometimes is not a linear progression. There are times when learning happens faster than normal, usually when judokas prepare for competitions and promotional exams. There are also times when the learning process reaches plateaus, which are normal and can be managed by temporarily switching attention to another area of judo, before coming back to the issue with a refreshed view. Injuries may also create setbacks in the process of learning judo. Accordingly, the color of the belt and the temporary levels of performance should not be as important in terms of the priorities of a judoka. A long-term vision in which judo is incorporated as part of a judoka's lifestyle, with perseverance, determination, and a continuous desire to learn, are significantly more important. Additional resources to learn more about judo from a broad perspective include the books by Inokuma and Sato (1986), and Nishioka and West (1979).

As in many other athletic activities, such as running or biking, there are inherent risks of injury when judo is conducted over an extended period of time. However, many injuries can be prevented, and when unavoidable, managed in a way that their impact is reduced. Knowledge of the risks is key in this process, particularly when it comes to basic diagnostics to identify high-risk situations that require the involvement of a healthcare professional. Regular training in first aid, cardiopulmonary resuscitation techniques (CPR), and the use of Automated External Defibrillator equipment (AED) are very valuable to know how to respond to health-related occurrences. The American Red Cross and the American Heart Association, among others, provide training in which people can become certified in first aid/CPR/AED. While judokas of all levels are encouraged to gain a decent knowledge of the medical issues surrounding the practice of judo, a good understanding of this topic is particularly necessary for instructors, coaches, and referees. The medical risks specifically associated with the practice of judo, and the ways to properly address them, are explained in a book about the medical care of the judoka by sports medicine expert Anthony Catanese (2012). A chapter addressing the medical issues frequently experienced by master judokas may be of particular interest to people over 30 years old.

Concussions represent an area of particular concern that judo practitioners should be aware of. Learning how to recognize the early signs and symptoms of possible concussions can make a big difference in the extent of the damage and the recovery process. The Centers for Disease Control and Prevention (CDC) offers free online training, such as the Heads Up course, which alerts people to the dangers of concussions. The Safe Sport course developed by the United States Olympic Committee also contributes to promoting a safe environment for judo athletes.

A general recommendation for avoiding injuries in the practice of judo is allocating enough time for warm-up exercises. As Nishioka explained, it is important to increase the body temperature in a gradual way and place particular emphasis in warming up those parts of the body that bend, twist and rotate, such as ankles, knees, elbows, wrists, shoulders, and the neck (2010: 144-5). Also important is the determination to reduce the intensity or stop participating in judo activities as soon as a potential injury is identified, regardless of what other people may say or think. Many injuries are worsened by continued practice when people should have already stopped, so it is preferable to take a break and have a faster recovery process. Overall, becoming knowledgeable about the health risks of participating in an athletic activity such as judo can go a long way in the process of preventing injuries and having a safer judo experience in general.

One important consideration is that judo techniques should not be used on people outside authorized settings, such the practice dojo, competitions, and official demonstrations. If used on people outside these settings, judo training may be interpreted as an unfair advantage, comparable to the use of a weapon. Even when judo practitioners need to defend themselves or others from physical aggression, the response should only be proportional to the threat.

At some point in the life of a judoka, if there is an opportunity to do so, it would be a rewarding experience to visit the Kodokan Judo Institute, currently located in the Bunkyo ward in Tokyo, Japan. The possibility of talking to the highly knowledgeable judo instructors of the Kodokan, and practice judo at its facilities, would be a unique experience. The Kodokan has an international department, whose staff can speak English and take reservations for visitors at the Kodokan hostel. At any given time, there are many judo practitioners of different ages and with different levels of skill coming from different parts of the world, who tend to communicate in English regardless of their country of origin. The instructors of the Kodokan at the randori class also speak English, which facilitates the communications.

The Kodokan offers visitors with enough level of skill to practice judo with black belts the opportunity to join its randori class. There are daily passes if one only stays for a few days. There are also kata classes available once a week on Tuesdays. The main requirement is to have a white judogi. If someone only wants to observe the judo practice, there is free access to the spectators' area on the top floor of the Kodokan building. Wednesdays are good for watching judo practice, because that day is when students from the university teams, including top-level competitors, go to practice at the Kodokan.

Learning about the life of Jigoro Kano, the founder of judo, is something every judoka should do. Beyond the little pieces of information about him, like the fact that his favorite technique was uki goshi, it is important to appreciate that the task of taking martial arts techniques intended to kill and injure, and turning them into an organized sequence of movements that are safe for people of all ages to practice, is a remarkable feat. The commitment he showed disseminating judo around the world, at a time where most international travel was done by ship, is nothing short of extraordinary. The persuasive writing style reflected in his letters is also worthy of admiration, as was his vision for judo practitioners to make use of their strength, skills and wisdom to both improve themselves and make positive contributions to society. The book on Jigoro Kano and his students, authored by martial arts authors John Stevens (2013), is a good way to learn about the original spirit of judo.

Learning about famous judo competitors and outstanding personalities in judo is another area that judokas should become familiar with. A few names of people whose careers should be reviewed include Yasuhiro Yamashita, Kyuzo Mifune, Isao Inokuma, Teddy Riner, Keiko Fukuda, Jimmy Takemori, Hayward Nishioka, James Bregman, Ben Nighthorse Campbell, Jimmy Pedro, Kayla Harrison, AnnMaria De Mars and Ronda Rousey. The emergence of Brazilian jiujitsu has also made it important to learn about the story of Royce Gracie and his relatives, among other representatives of this discipline.

The way forward should be defined by perseverance and dedication to continue learning about the different dimensions of judo. When you welcome judo as part of your life, it can give you long-term rewards, helping you achieve a way of life that promotes physical and mental harmony, contributing to a balanced lifestyle, and ultimately encouraging you to make positive contributions to society.

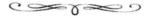

Thank you for reading this book to the end. If you found the information contained in this book helpful, then please consider leaving a review. As an author, I place great value on the feedback provided by readers, even if it is just a few words. Your thoughts and impressions about the book may help others benefit from the content provided in these pages as well. You may enter your comments on the website of the bookstore where you acquired this book.

Glossary

Glossary

Judo Uniform

Judogi	=	Judo uniform
Obi	=	Belt
Uwagi	=	Judo jacket
Shitagi	=	Judo pants
Sode	=	Sleeve
Eri	=	Lapel
Zori	=	Slippers

Greetings and Positions

Rei	=	Bow
Ritsurei	=	Standing bow
Seiza	=	Sit in a kneeling position
Zarei	=	Kneeling bow
Anza	=	Sitting cross-legged
Kiotsuke	=	Attention, get ready
Shomen-ni rei	=	Bow to the founder of judo
Sensei-ni rei	=	Bow to sensei

Parts of a Throw

Kumi kata	=	Establishing a grip
Kuzushi	=	Getting partner off balance
Tsukuri	=	Positioning for a throw
Kake	=	Executing a throw

Definitions and Principles

Judo	=	The gentle way
Budo	=	Practice of the martial way
Bushido	=	Way of life of the samurai
Jita kyoei	=	Mutual benefit for welfare
Seryonku zenyo	=	Maximum efficiency with minimal effort

Competition Scores

Ippon	=	Full point, instant win
Wazari	=	Score, half a point
Yuko	=	Score, less than a wazari
Wazari awazete ippon	=	Ippon by two wazari

Referee Calls

Hajime	=	Begin
Matte	=	Stop
Osaekomi	=	Start hold-down count
Toketa	=	Stop the hold-down count
Sore made	=	Time is up, that is all
Shido	=	Minor penalty
Hansoku make	=	Major penalty
Hantei	=	Call for judges' decision
Sono mama	=	Freeze, do not move
Yoshi	=	Restart after freezing
Fusen gachi	=	Win by default
Kiken gachi	=	Win by injury, inability or withdrawal of opponent
Yusei gachi	=	Win by referee's decision
Hiki waki	=	Even match, draw

Activities

Randori	=	Free sparring practice
Ukemi	=	Breakfall
Zempo kaiten	=	Forward rolling breakfall
Mokuso	=	Meditate
Kata	=	Prearranged techniques
Uchi komi	=	Repetitive techniques
Shiai	=	Judo tournament
Hokaku shiai	=	The winner remains
Batsugun	=	Instant promotion
Kappo	=	Method of resuscitation

Parts of the Body

Te	=	Hand
Ude	=	Arm
Hiji	=	Elbow
Wake	=	Armpit
Hara	=	Stomach
Koshi, Goshi	=	Hip
Ashi	=	Foot or leg
Hiza	=	Knee

Body Movement

Shisei	=	Posture
Shizentai	=	Natural posture
Jigotai	=	Defensive posture
Shintai	=	Body movement
Ayumi ashi	=	Natural walking
Tsugi ashi	=	One foot after the other
Tai sabaki	=	Slipping movement

Groups of Techniques

Nage waza	=	Throwing techniques
Tachi waza	=	Standing techniques
Ne waza	=	Matwork techniques
Katame waza	=	Grappling techniques
Osaekomi waza	=	Holding techniques
Shime waza	=	Choking techniques
Kansetsu waza	=	Armbar techniques
Renraku waza	=	Combinations
Kaeshi waza	=	Counterattack techniques
Tokui waza	=	Favorite techniques
Atemi waza	=	Striking techniques
Sutemi waza	=	Sacrifice techniques

Actions and Qualifiers

Guruma	=	Wheel
Barai, Harai	=	Sweep
Gari	=	Reap
Gake	=	Hook
O	=	Major, Large
Ko	=	Minor, Small
Otoshi	=	Drop
Soto	=	Outer
Uchi	=	Inner

Directions

Mae	=	Front
Yoko	=	Side
Ushiro	=	Back
Migi	=	Right
Hidari	=	Left

People

Kyoshi	=	Instructor
Sensei	=	Head or senior instructor
Shihan	=	Model teacher (i.e. Kano)
Judoka	=	Judo practitioner
Mudansha	=	Judokas without a black belt
Yudansha	=	Judokas with a black belt
Kodansha	=	High-ranking judokas
Tori	=	Person applying technique
Uke	=	Person receiving technique
Shimpan	=	Referee

Places

Dojo	=	Martial arts center
Joseki	=	Side for senior officials
Tatami	=	Surface to practice judo
Kodokan	=	Judo institute in Japan

Numbers

Ichi	=	One
Ni	=	Two
San	=	Three
Shi	=	Four
Go	=	Five
Roku	=	Six
Shichi	=	Seven
Hachi	=	Eight
Ku	=	Nine
Ju	=	Ten
Ju ichi	=	Eleven
Ni ju	=	Twenty

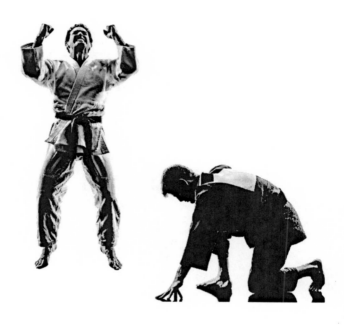

*Competitions are valuable, but winning at all costs
should not be the goal of judo practice*

References

References

Catanese, Anthony
2012   The Medical Care of the Judoka: A Guide for Athletes, Coaches and Referees to Common Medical Problems in Judo. Wheatmark. Tucson, Arizona.

De Mars, AnnMaria and James Pedro Sr.
2013   Winning on the Ground: Training and Techniques for Judo and MMA Fighters. Black Belt Books. Valencia, California.

Ferguson, Rhadi
2014   The Ultimate Judo Success Secret. Electronic book, Rhadi Ferguson.

Figueroa, Nestor
2004   Pedagogía del Judo. Electronic book, Sinchijudokan Institute.

Hernandez, Israel
2015   Everything you Should Know about Uchi Mata. Isvael Sport / Flores Productions. DVD video.

Inokuma, Isao and Nobuyuki Sato
1986   Best Judo. Kodansha International. New York.

Imada, Vaughn, David Matsumoto, Joon Chi, Karen Mackey, Dean Markovics, Bryan Matsuoka, Chris Mitsuoka, Ann Marie Rousey, and Eiko Shepherd
2004   The Psychological and Behavioral Effects of Judo. White paper, United States Judo Federation. 12 pages.

Kano, Jigoro
2013   Kodokan Judo. Kodansha USA. New York.

Matsumoto, David
2003   The Light of Kodokan Judo: Essays on Judo and Judo Instruction in Japan. Electronic resource, United States Judo Federation. Accessed on 7/20/2015. http://www.usjf.com/wp-content/uploads/2013/08/compilation.pdf

Morley, Gary and Leila Hussain
2015   Kosovo's Judo Queen Fights for Recognition. Electronic resource. Acc. on 8/5/2015. http://edition.cnn.com/2015/06/17/sport/majlinda-kelmendi-kosovo-judo-olympics

Nishioka, Hayward
2000   Judo: Heart and Soul. Black Belt Books. Valencia, California.
2010   Training for Competition: Judo Coaching, Strategy and the Science for Success. Black Belt Books. Valencia, California.

Nishioka, Hayward and James West
1979   The Judo Textbook: In Practical Application. Black Belt Books. Valencia, California.

Ohlenkamp, Neil
S/D   What Does a Judo Black Belt Really Mean? Electronic resource, Judoinfo. Acc. on 10/15/2015. http://judoinfo.com/bb.htm

Otaki, Tadao and Donn Draeger
1983   Judo Formal Techniques: A Complete Guide to Kodokan Randori no Kata. Tuttle Martial Arts. North Clarendon, Vermont.

Thompson, George and Jerry Jenkins
2013   Verbal Judo: The Gentle Art of Persuasion. HarperCollins Books. New York.

Panasonic
2015   Business Philosophy. Electronic resource. Accessed on 8/5/2015. http://www.panasonic.com/ global/ corporate/management/philosophy.html

Pedro, Jimmy
2007   Grip Like a World Champion. DVD Video.

Ravizza, Ken and Tom Hanson
1998   Heads-Up Baseball: Playing the Game One Pitch at a Time. Masters Press. Chicago, Illinois.

Rousey, Ronda
2015   My Fight / Your Fight. Regan Arts. New York.

Stevens, John
2013   The Way of Judo: A Portrait of Jigoro Kano and His Students. Shambhala Publications. Boston, Massachusetts.

Watanabe, Jiichi and Lindy Avakian
1990   The Secrets of Judo: A Text for Instructors and Students. Tuttle Publishing. North Clarendon, Vermont.

Recommended Resources

In this book, many important subjects were only covered in a superficial way. The following list includes the top seven resources I would recommend for judo practitioners interested in learning more about judo.

1. Kodokan Judo. Jigoro Kano (2013). Kodansha USA. New York.

2. Judo: Heart and Soul. Haywayd Nishioka (2000). Black Belt Books. Valencia, California.

3. Winning on the Ground: Training and Techniques for Judo and MMA Fighters. AnnMaria De Mars and James Pedro (2013). Black Belt Books. Valencia, California.

4. Judo Formal Techniques: A Complete Guide to Kodokan Randori no Kata. Tadao Otaki and Donn Draeger (1983). Tuttle Martial Arts. North Clarendon, Vermont.

5. The Medical Care of the Judoka: A Guide for Athletes, Coaches and Referees to Common Medical Problems in Judo. Anthony Catanese (2012). Wheatmark. Tucson, Arizona.

6. Grip Like a World Champion. Jimmy Pedro (2007). DVD video.

7. Everything you Should Know about Uchi Mata. Israel Hernandez (2015). DVD video.

Acknowledgements

I would like to express my gratitude to my judo instructors, who helped me at different stages in my judo learning process: Ricardo Inami, Jorge Miranda, Luis Bonilla, and Michael and Sharon Landstreet. Special thanks to Gaiv Tata, Robert Winston and John Morrison as well. I also benefited from the encouragement and advice provided by members of Shufu Yudanshakai. Big thanks to my judo comrades as well, who made the practice of judo possible.

I would also like to thank Hayward Nishioka and Charles Medani, who reviewed the draft version of this manuscript and provided very valuable suggestions. The feedback provided by Christopher Compton, Patrick Ramsey and Benjamin Lee was of great consequence as well. I am also grateful for the continued support of my family.

As an author, writing this book was a very fulfilling experience. I am thankful for the opportunity to reflect on the issues surrounding the practice of judo, and I hope beginner judokas find it useful in their judo paths.

About the Author

Rodolfo Tello is a black belt judo practitioner currently based in Arlington, Virginia. He started doing judo more than twenty years ago and is still active in regular judo practice. He is a Certified National Coach in judo and is also certified as a judo referee. He is a life member of the United States Judo Federation and is affiliated with Shufu Yudanshakai, the black belt association of the Mid-Atlantic region of the United States. He is also a cultural anthropologist with a PhD from American University and a master's degree from the University of Maryland.

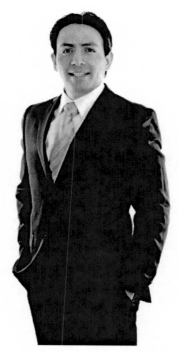

Additional information about the author and his publications may be found at www.rodolfotello.com

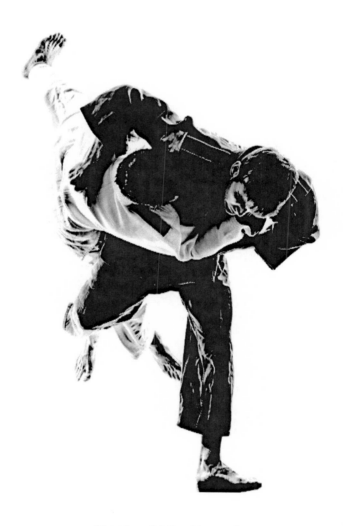

Harai goshi (koshi waza)

CPSIA information can be obtained at www.ICGtesting.com
Printed in the USA
LVOW10s1516040816

499078LV00001B/70/P

9 781633 870017